FUNDAMENTAL ASSUMPTION FOR STRONG RELATIONSHIP

Building Enduring Love

Manuela A.Sigel

ABOUT THE BOOK

Find the groundbreaking force of cognizant presumptions in "Fundamental Assumption for Strong Relationship" Plunge into an excursion of trust, sympathy, and immovable responsibility, disclosing the crucial convictions that support persevering through associations. Investigate the way to supporting significant love, shared regard, and enduring concordance — an outline for building connections that flourish. Embrace the ethos of figuring out, thoughtfulness, and significant association as you explore the delightful intricacies of organization. Lift your associations with the core values that structure solid, enduring bonds. Open the key to making a groundwork of affection and trust that goes the distance.

ABOUT THE AUTHOR

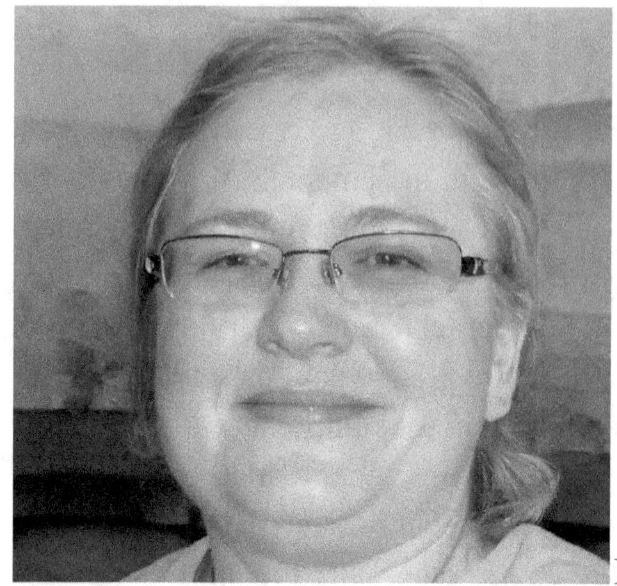

Meet the splendid psyche behind "Fundamental Assumption for Strong Relationship" the regarded creator Manuela A. Sigel. Pulling in an energy for investigating the complexities of human association, Manuela brings an abundance of shrewdness and skill to the domain of relationship elements and self-improvement.

With a foundation in brain science and a well established obligation to enabling people as they continued looking for significant associations,

Manuela's excursion as a creator has been portrayed by a devotion to unwinding the intricacies of human connections. Her sagacious perceptions and sympathetic methodology have reverberated with perusers around the world, offering them significant experiences and groundbreaking systems to develop persevering and satisfying organizations.

Known for her merciful nature and enduring confidence in the force of understanding and sympathy, Manuela's work rises above simple words on a page — it fills in as a directing light for people looking to explore the difficulties of associations with effortlessness and legitimacy. Her interesting point of view and significant comprehension of the human mind implant each page of "Fundamental Assumption for Strong Relationship" with intelligence, pragmatic counsel, and a profound love for the extraordinary capability of cognizant association.

As an idea chief in the field of relationship brain research, Manuela's effect stretches out a long way past the pages of her book. Through her composition, talking commitment, and training attempts, she proceeds to motivate and enable people to cultivate connections grounded in trust, regard, and unrestricted love.

Join Manuela on an excursion of self-disclosure, development, and significant association as she welcomes you to investigate the principal suspicions that support solid and persevering through connections. Her direction and mastery prepare for perusers to leave on an extraordinary way towards building satisfying and significant associations that go the distance.

In the possession of Manuela A. Sigel, "Fundamental Assumption for Strong Relationship" isn't simply a book — it's an encouraging sign, a guide to profound and enduring association, and a demonstration of the extraordinary force of cognizant, purposeful connections

TABLE OF CONTENT

INTRODUCTION

INTRODUCTION

What makes a relationship work?

A happy relationship is made possible by a variety of factors, including; Love, commitment, trust, time, attention, good communication, including listening, partnership, tolerance, patience, openness, honesty, respect, sharing, consideration, generosity, willingness/ability to compromise, constructive management of disagreements/arguments, willingness to see another person's point of view, ability and willingness to forgive/apologize, and fun are all qualities that are essential. The rundown is basic and self-evident yet it tends to be extremely challenging for people/couples to reestablish their relationship to a delightful one when troubles emerge or when they float separated.

There are many areas of closeness that can help a marriage or relationship stay strong, improve, and get back on track when it has become distant or difficult. Some of the time couples feel that things are not right between them, they can't help thinking about what's going on and what they can do?

The accompanying four areas of closeness can assist with directing a couple in evaluating how their relationship is and can likewise direct a couple in how to turn out to be nearer and further develop their relationship when challenges emerge, or when they have become far off from each other.

Areas of Closeness
Doing things Together:Actual Closeness
Profound Closeness:Sexual Closeness

None of the four regions above are a higher priority than one another yet each can assist one more region with flourishing and all together they can assist a relationship with turning out to be really fulfilling, closer, more private

Doing Things Together

Couples should get to know one another. With occupied lives, numerous responsibilities and kids to really focus on couples can wind up with next to no time for one another. Regular outings like shopping, dining out, going to the movies, walking, swimming, participating in sports, exercising, sharing hobbies, and going on vacations can help couples get to know one another better and spend more time together.

Actual Closeness

A couple really should be close truly. This can incorporate eye to eye connection, clasping hands, embracing, sitting near one another, rubbing each other. More open doors for actual closeness will improve a couple's feeling of closeness and closeness. Couples need to be aware that some people are more comfortable being physically demonstrative than others. It's also important to try to figure out how comfortable your partner is and work from there.

Profound Closeness

Profound closeness will assist couples with getting to be aware and see each other all the more profoundly and furthermore have sympathy for one another. It includes opening up to one another about sentiments, contemplations, convictions, values, trusts, stresses, fears, dreams and desires. Mindful listening upgrades profound closeness when the two people tune in to get to be aware and grasp their companion/accomplice all the more completely, as opposed to dissent, judge, fault or censure their mate/accomplice.

Sexual closeness

It is essential that both partners are content with their sexual relationship and feel comfortable raising and discussing it whenever necessary. Once in a while couples can be exceptionally worried about the recurrence of their sexual movement. However long the two people are content with the recurrence and the idea of their sexual movement there is no requirement for them to be concerned or to contrast their sexual relationship with those depicted in the media or those detailed by others of their associate, the two of which can be at odds with the real world.

Chapter 1: The Heart of Maturity in Love.

To be able to do genuine love implies becoming full grown, with reasonable assumptions for the other individual. It implies tolerating liability regarding our own bliss or despondency, and neither anticipating that the other individual should fulfill us nor faulting that individual for our terrible temperaments and dissatisfactions.

Development, by and large, is numerous things. Development in an affectionate relationship is everything! To begin with, it is the capacity to base a choice about an affection relationship on the higher perspective - the long stretch. As a rule, it implies having the option to miss the diversion for the second and select the game-plan which will pay off later.

In an affection relationship, it implies having the option to partake in the moment delight that accompanies the sentiment existing apart from everything else while realizing the best is yet to be and showing restraint while you watch your affection develop.

Knowing by cooperating, the condition of genuine love will introduce itself in the relationship and will develop with time. It is realizing that you develop into an adoration relationship. It doesn't occur at the same time. Mature love accomplices look for better approaches to help each other develop.

One of the attributes of early stages is the "I need it currently" approach. Grown-up individuals can pause. What's more, frequently they don't. Frequently they permit themselves to slip once again into outset so they can legitimize racing into things.

Development is the capacity to stay with a task or a circumstance until it is done. It implies taking the necessary steps to cause the relationship to be one you are pleased to be in. The grown-up who is continually evolving position, connections, and companions, is in a word. . . youthful. They can't stick it out on the grounds that they are not adults. Everything inevitably appears to go bad.

Note. . . For an affectionate relationship to develop, the two accomplices should encounter a profound inclination, an implied conviction, that something really stands out about them which couldn't have ever happened had each not added to its creation.

Mature love accomplices have learned not to expect flawlessness in one another. They realize that acknowledgement has its own prize. Every darling's disparities test the other's ability for acknowledgment, absolution and understanding. They never dance around issues.

At the point when it is important, they talk about their defects, affectionately, with care not to condemn with hurtful words. Acknowledgment and resistance clasp hands within the sight of unqualified love.

Mature sweethearts - - darlings who love genuinely - - foster a skill for evading disdain and zeroing in on the great they find in each other. They have developed to a more elevated level of understanding, one that rises above considering the blemishes of the other.
Development is the ability to confront repulsiveness, disappointment, inconvenience and rout without grievance or breakdown. Mature love accomplices realize they can't have everything in their own specific manner. They can concede to conditions, to others - and to time, when fundamental.

Mature love accomplices license each other the opportunity to seek after their singular advantages and companions without limitation. This is when trust introduces itself. Mature love permits this degree of separateness to unite sweethearts. In this situation separateness is seen as a security, not a wedge. It urges love accomplices to commend their own uniqueness.

Note. . . we can come to understand that full grown love approaches adoring yourself for being what you are, and similarly cherishing someone else for what their identity is. At the point when we can feel such unqualified regardless of how-you-act love, we have realized what I call mature love. Mature love permits you completely to act naturally with your adored one.

Development is the capacity to satisfy the obligations of an affectionate relationship, and this implies being trustworthy.

It implies keeping your promise; it implies living in your relationship like your assertion truly implies something. Steadfastness likens with individual trustworthiness.

This implies no holds back. It implies getting out whatever should be said, with affection. Are you really serious about what you say? Do you express whatever you might be thinking?

The world is loaded up with individuals who can't be depended on, individuals who never appear to follow through in the grip, individuals who break commitments and substitute explanations for execution. They rationalize. They appear late - or not by any stretch of the imagination. They are confused and disarranged. Their lives are a tumultuous labyrinth of incomplete business and uncertain connections. Gracious, what a tangled web we weave.

Note. . . Mature love offers us our most significant chance for recovering completeness - not on the grounds that our accomplices will fill the entirety of our void, but since we can utilize the hug of a caring relationship to sustain ourselves toward more prominent development and aging.

Development is the capacity to go with a choice and stand by it. Youthful individuals spend their lives investigating vast potential outcomes and afterward sit idle. Activity requires fortitude. There is no development without boldness.

Development is the capacity to saddle your capacities and your energies and to accomplish more than is normal in your connections. The full grown individual will not make due with unremarkableness. They would prefer to reach skyward and come up short than point low and hit it.

Living by Adoration Morals.

A relationship is all about infusing every part of your partnership with deep respect, empathy, and authentic love. When you live by adoring morals, it means you deeply honor and cherish your partner, and you both constantly work to understand and support each other.

Open, honest communication is crucial. It's about creating a safe space where both of you can freely express your feelings, thoughts, and fears, knowing that you'll always have each other's understanding and respect. This kind of communication helps you navigate your differences, dream together, and build a future based on shared values and goals.

Respecting each other's individual space and boundaries is also so important. It means that you both empower and support each other's personal growth and passions without trying to change or control one another. It's about being independent individuals who cherish and complement each other.

Living by adoration morals also includes a commitment to personal reflection and growth. It's about recognizing your impact on the relationship, being open to feedback, and striving to become the best partner you can be. This approach ensures that both of you are contributing to the relationship's health and happiness, fostering a space where you both can learn and grow together.

At its core, living by adoration morals is about understanding that love is an active, ongoing practice. It's a commitment to consistently honor and cherish your partner, to respect and care for each other every day.

A timeless foundation for building a deep, purposeful connection. It's an intentional, transformative approach to partnership that thrives on principles like respect, empathy, and unwavering commitment. By embracing adoration morals, you build a relationship full of harmony, support, and enduring love—a relationship grounded in deep respect and unwavering care for each other.

Chapter 2: Nurturing Friendship.

Companion is just characterized as "a like "an individual and appreciate being with," and Closest companion as "one's nearest and closest companion."

Companions have comparable interests and closest companions even offer the delights and distresses of life.

Having your companion as your dearest companion can be one of the extraordinary advantages of marriage. Assuming you and your mate are now closest companions, that is superb; on the off chance that not, perhaps now is the right time to grasp the significance of fellowship in marriage.

Kinship is one of the qualities of a cheerful and enduring marriage, as well as the groundwork of a sound marriage.

Research has shown that couples that have an incredible companionship have a higher rate by and large of conjugal fulfillment. As a matter of fact, the close to home association that married couples share is supposed to be multiple times more significant than their actual closeness. Couples that are companions anticipate getting to know each other, and truly like each other.

Their exercises and interests really become upgraded in light of the fact that they have their number one individual with whom to share their background.

Constructing and supporting the conjugal kinship can reinforce a marriage since fellowship in marriage is known to fabricate profound and actual closeness. Fellowship assists wedded couples with having a solid sense of security enough to be more open with each other without stressing over being judged or feeling unreliable.

Sustaining and constructing that companionship in marriage requires practice and takes time and exertion. The following are some conjugal companionship building abilities and methods to help maintain and reinforce your marriage.

Conjugal Fellowship Building:

- **Time:** Hang out

- **Correspondence:** Talk and offer about regular day to day existence

- **Trust:** tell the truth and faithful

- **Interests:** Find normal interests Play around with each other. Snicker together Gain enduring experiences Do and attempt new things together

- **Objectives:** Put forth and work towards life objectives with each other. Dream together

- **Need:** Focus on your life partner. Feel like Regards each other Treat each other similarly Cheer on one another's victories Rest on each other in the midst of hardship. Value your mate Be thoughtful of one another Be pardoning of each other don't hold hard feelings.

Realizing your companion well is a critical component in becoming or staying dearest companions with your accomplice. Playing "get to know you" or "self random data" games can be a really supportive and fun activity. Test each other on subtleties, for example, name of your primary school, your blood classification, main tune, or greatest turn on. Make the award something like: who does family errands, foot or back rubs, or the champ will pick the following film or café.

Actual closeness might blur in a marriage,but the profound closeness needn't. Genuine kinship endures forever.

What Style My Partner Adopts.

The most effective method to Figure out Your Accomplice's Takes on Style

Does it seem like you and your accomplice are never in total agreement? Maybe you accept your style?

an accomplice is unapproachable, penniless, envious or free and maybe their attributes are the direct inverse of yours. The explanation might be that you and your accomplice have different connection styles. Nonetheless, by understanding your accomplice's connection style, you can track down better ways of dealing with your relationship.

All in all, what is your accomplice ?

Accomplice's Styles

There are four fundamental accomplice's styles. These are; secure, restless distracted, pretentious avoidant and unfortunate avoidant.

56% of the populace are secure

- 20% of individuals have a restless connection style

- 23% are avoidant

- 1% are unfortunate avoidant.

Are Accomplices Embracing Styles Undesirable?

It is essential to take note that you can't class different accomplice's styles as solid or unfortunate. These styles all exist for an explanation, and they are there to assist individuals with exploring connections. Thus, prior to deciding your accomplice's style, make sure to relinquish any judgment.

A connection style isn't something that necessities fixing. Notwithstanding, by perceiving your accomplice's embrace style, you can start to comprehend your accomplice on a more profound level to ensure your relationship is as great as could be expected.

Key accomplice's Style Qualities

Secure56% of individuals will show a protected connection style. These individuals normally have an elevated degree of the capacity to understand people on a deeper level and will have a helpful approach to showing their feelings. A few vital characteristics for individuals with a safe accomplice's style are;

- Sets solid and sensible limits
- Feels similarly great alone and with an accomplice
- Has a positive view on connections
- Shows versatility, with a capacity to lament, learn and continue on
- Glad to examine issues to tackle issues

Restless Distracted

20% of individuals have this as their essential connection style. With this, these people will normally have a more apprehensive outlook on connections and perhaps less secure in their connections. A few normal characteristics with this embrace style incorporate;

- May have programmed negative reasoning - promptly jumping to the most pessimistic scenario translation

- Battles with being separated from everyone else, and will frequently require approval from an accomplice to have a good sense of reassurance

- May battle with relationship stressors, for example, envy, oversensitivity, poverty and emotional episodes.

Contemptuous Avoidant

This embraced style will remain closely connected with those you might depict as having developed a wall. The 23% that have this style will regularly be exceptionally independent and independent. Thus, they might battle to give anybody access. Different characteristics incorporate;

- Avoiding the chance rely upon others or have wards
- Feels more open to having colleagues than cozy connections
- May appear to be detached forceful during conflicts

- Normally prefers to be truly and sincerely far off and may drive individuals away when they get excessively close.

Unfortunate Avoidant

Normally, only 1% of individuals partner with this style. With unfortunate avoidant (otherwise called restless avoidant) these people might have not very many truly cozy connections and will feel awkward drawing near to other people. Key attributes might show as;

- Battles with an internal clash around closeness

- Doesn't depend on others and will lack trust in others
- May fear private circumstances and be dubious of others' aims.

Step by step instructions to Decide Your Accomplice's taken on Style

While we can never truly know how an accomplice is feeling where it counts, there as a few key markers that can assist you with deciding your accomplice's style;

Check Your Discussions out
At the point when your accomplice talks, are they;

- Simple organization and feels free and happy with discussing a scope of subjects, including themselves and their sentiments.
- Awkward discussing sentiments and spotlights on what they do instead of what they feel or what their identity is.
- Appears to be truly certain and connecting with and extremely anxious to please and make the discussion as agreeable as could be expected.

How Would They Discuss Themselves?

When your accomplice self-unveils, what occurs?

- They find overseeing strain well and will be perky and ready to self-unveil individual data.
- Your accomplice is probably not going to discuss their internal identity and would feel awkward self-uncovering.
- They are probably going to unveil excessively, too early. It might seem to be over-enthusiastic as they need to find closeness rapidly.

Their Dating History

What does your accomplice's dating history resemble?

- Your accomplice has had a couple of committed relationships yet has likewise had timeframes alone.
- They might not have had any committed relationships previously, bound to have

> dated a great deal, yet not settled with anybody for any period of time.
> - Your accomplice has had a progression of accomplices, both long and momentary associations with very little time alone.

On the off chance that your accomplice is fundamentally 1s — This is probably going to show that your accomplice has a solid connection style.

Predominantly 2s — This shows an avoidant connection style, where they are commonly independent and rather not get excessively close.

For mostly 3s — Your accomplice is showing a restless connection style, where they might battle with security in the relationship.

Help! We Have Different Takes on Styles!

It is normal for accomplices to have different embraced styles, and on the off chance that you and your accomplice's styles are unique, this doesn't mean your relationship is ill-fated. Nonetheless, by seeing each other's embraced type and doing whatever it takes to know about a portion of the signs of the taken on style, it becomes simpler to explore relationship hardships.

Chapter 3: Responding to Your Partner's Feelings.

Defend/ Get a handle on

A commonplace fashion for excusing a tendency is to cover or represent yourself after your mate tells you how the person being pertained to feels. The effect is to look at how you feel and to miss how your mate feels.

The explanation I said." What I suggested was.

Apologize

Explanations of disappointment offered unnecessarily hot before you let your soul mate in on that you sound the passions that were participated regularly sum to nothing. They really aggregate to the communication" I would prefer not to dissect this farther and I would authentically rather not hear how seriously I hurt you. Perhaps a quick placatory opinion will end this horrendous discussion."

still, admit my expressions of guilt that" I should not have said that "

If it's not too much trouble.

Attack

Still, enlightening her when she makes you feel terrible is an unpretentious yet veritable and squashing Attack, If your mate tells you when you made her vibe horrendous. The result will be either a long and warmed series of counterassaults or a retreat into cold quietness.

" I yield what I did was deceived, yet you" In light of everything, perhaps you are right, but what I can not sound is the explanation you.

Advice

Right when your life abettor shares a weight or fight, do not incontinently offer Direction. The deflected life mate demanded the help of a partner who admired him, not the contemplations of an assistant who allowed He demanded" help." Laid back women regularly offer directions to disturb misters, not understanding that the communication their misters hear is" Tune in, you sissy, I will tell you how to manage this, since you are not kidding!"

" Perhaps you should " " It seems to me that if you.

misprision

Right when your associate offers a tendency, norway misprision- telling the existent being pertained to not to feel" like that.`` Anyhow, when you're trying to help, to enlighten someone not to witness an inclination the existent has as of late conveyed much of the time is by all accounts a putdown. rulings like " Honey, you should not feel consequently" or" There is no great reason to feel so anxious(hurt, etc)" should be avoided.

" I do not really see the provocation behind why you feel.." Indeed, honey, there is a satisfying explanation I need to feel..

Right

Another reasonable yet unpretentious system for excusing opinions is to address a singular's evaluation of the issue that's making a tendency. To tell the singular what the issue" really is' ' and what the existent being pertained to should in this manner sense does not bestow protestation. In the long run, it may be critical to suggest an exact perspective on events, yet to do so following a tendency is communicated conveys excusal

" What I suppose you authentically mean is." I do not suppose you feel..

Approaches to enduring Opinions

- **Reflecting the tendency back like a glass"** maybe you feel"" Assume you authentically felt.. when.

- **Make sense of by depicting what you heard and curious with respects to whether you heard rightly."** Are you saying that..." I continue to consider whether you feel.

- **Explore what was suggested by asking questions."** I am doubtful what you mean" When do you feel differently? I do not precisely understand how you feel about..

- **Connect by suggesting colorful opinions that are associated with what has been participated."** You really felt... Did you also feel..." I can see that you feel.. still, I could in like manner sense, If I ever happened to fantasize being in your circumstance.. Do you feel like that?"

Work out

Bit by bit directions to Answer When Your associate Offers passions Worksheet

One of the most inconvenient yet huge capacities to make is the capability to help our assistants with feeling honored when they partake in a tendency with us. A critical number of us have hardly any familiarity with the multitudinous ways we convey examination or bias or heartlessness when our mates express their opinions.

Whenever we answer antagonistically, our mates feel hurt and seek sanctum behind anything that cloak shields them from redundant hurt. This exercise is planned to help you with sorting out some way to answer your life abettor 's opinions to such an extent that will construct a sensation of warmth, understanding, and closeness.

Right when your adjunct tells you how the existent feels, you ought to treat that tendency with care. Review that when someone really recognizes your opinions, you'll in and large sense appreciated and admired and you're inclined to partake your own special further noteworthy sum opinions.

Shared objectives and dreams.

Defining Objects can be a useful cycle for individuals who are hoping to make progressions in their lives. This strategy for responsibility can likewise incorporate couples who are in a solid, forward- moving relationship that they wish to keep and work on together later on.

Assuming you are reticent to put forth objects with your soul mate or neglect to see the point, seeing precisely why dating objects are significant could help with giving simplicity and bearing that could ameliorate your particular satisfaction together.

The following, we are probing the advantages you can appreciate from putting two or three objects, as well as what objects you might suppose about setting in a relationship. We will likewise be diving into how to lay out objects, uniting you to colorful systems to help you with taking advantage of your experience.

Why Are cohorts objects Sound?

Putting forth objects with your life mate can be a system for guaranteeing that you're in total agreement. It can likewise be a system to design the future and plan how you'll both arrive together.

objects can be salutary to use inside a relationship, as it by and large permits the two cohorts to convey their musts and inclinations. It also implies that the two people anticipate working on the relationship, conceivably making the relationship more.

What Is A Sound Organization?

Characterizing a sound relationship constantly boils down to every existent's singular experience and perceptiveness. Notwithstanding, numerous settle on specific rates that can be available seeing someone it to be considered healthy. These can include:

- Correspondence
- Shared regard
- Trust
- Genuineness
- Shared care and backing

What Objects Are Stylish In A Sound Organization?

numerous concur that the stylish objects to set in a sound association are bones
that plan to work on the relationship for all gatherings included. objects connecting with correspondence, independence inside the relationship, trust and fictitiousness are numerous times the bones that can make a relationship more. There are incontrovertibly

more cases of objects for a solid association too, like financial and close to home objects.

Defining objects can be a useful original step. Notwithstanding, all individualities from a relationship might encounter a more serious position of social fulfillment when they start to deal with them together. A solid original step could be recording your objects some place where you'll reliably see them — keeping them front of psyche. You may likewise consider examining dates, achievements and progress with your abettor to work with open correspondence and development as you push ahead together.

Making Shrewd objects and dreams

Creating shrewd objects is not simply smart in the conventional sense. The condensation represents specific factors that veritably much erected objects constantly have, constantly assuming a part in their substance.

We have added up the factors of a smart ideal beneath, by and large a Shrewd ideal is:

unequivocal

Being unequivocal in several objects might help you with deciding precisely the exact thing that you and your abettor need to achieve. rather than wide, foggy objects, you can decide to fix effects similar in particular that you and your abettor can also effectively decide the vital stages to negotiate them. On the off chance that your ideal can be stalled into a lower ideal, for case, it veritably well may be exorbitantly wide.

Quantifiable

To decide whether an ideal is quantifiable, you might ask yourself a solitary inquiry: " What tells you and your better half that your ideal has been achieved?" Making an objective quantifiable can make it simpler to follow, advance and fete it, which can give you both alleviation to go on in your cycle.

Doable

Putting forth incomprehensible objects can be adverse to your relationship and your cerebral heartiness, as you might encounter disappointment on the off chance that you neglect to achieve them. That's the reason numerous people decide to define attainable and more sensible objects. Doing so conceivably builds your openings for progress while relieving your adventure for disappointment and can be a conclusive instrument — giving you the inclination that what you need is simply accessible.

Important

As you plan your ideal, you should seriously consider asking yourself" Is the objective applicable to your relationship?" Knowing why you're defining this ideal and how it'll help your relationship can tell you and your life mate on the off chance that it's really important and may impact your alleviation emphatically going ahead.

Time- confined

Despite the fact that putting forth objects without an end date gives you a lot of occasion to negotiate them, it may not be as propelling you or your a bettor — conceivably making it harder to achieve the objects you've set. You might consider marking the timetable or time span that tells you and the other existent in the relationship when to cover your ideal's advancement.

Chapter 4: Give Love Words.

The most effective system to express adored words.

- Talk truly from your heart and express sympathy.
- conduct a particular effect you value that your abettor does.
- Tell your partner you love him /her habitually.
- shoot an in anticipated love letter or Post a fast note with significant communication.
- Offer inspirational statements.

For this situation, words are everything.Actions express stronger than words — if, obviously, your abettor 's adoration word is" encouraging statements." Whether they're composed or spoken, an individual whose adoration word is uplifting statements will put a great deal of significance on what they need to say.

Your words will say a lot, in any event, when you need to simply allow effects to go unnoticed. As a matter of fact, it's normal for introductory expressions like" I am thankful for." and" I love the way you." will go relatively far in conveying the quantum they're valued.

Your abettor will particularly see the value in praises, sincere thank you's, manually written notes, and hearing what they mean to other people. The ideal is to tell your abettor the quantum you mean to and the quantum you give it an alternate study.

What Are Encouraging statements?

Uplifting statements are the most extensively honored way to express affection, defeating quality time and demonstrations of administration. It also is the main love word that spins around verbal articulation.

Encouraging statements are words that conduct your affection, appreciation, and regard for one furtherperson.They are positive words and expressions used to inspire notoriety.

cohorts who give and receive love through uplifting statements will generally be a relationship who notice and watch about the craft of their lives. For illustration, they might be quick to see their abettor 's new hair style.

Cases of Encouraging statements

The following are a couple of cases of encouraging statements

" Everything's better when you are then."

" I feel a debt of gratitude when you."

" I was unfit to do this without you."

" I truly love the new outfit. It looks perfect on you!"

" I am so fortunate to accompany you."

" I am so appreciative to have you in my life."

" It dazed me when you."

" important thanks to you for."

" You're doing really inconceivable work. I am truly glad for you.

" You're so special to me."

" You're fabulous."

" Your assistance infers such an incredible quantum to me."

" You are joking!"

Advantages of Encouraging statements

Exercising encouraging statements really will in general put a lot of significance on what their abettor says, hearing encouraging statements can help band together with feeling recognized, fulfilled, and more joyous in a relationship.

By involving uplifting statements in your relationship, you're fortifying Correspondence among you and your abettor . You're showing your abettor that you notice and value them. At the point when your abettor feels appreciated, they're presumably going to encounter a more profound fulfillment with themselves and with the relationship.

Getting encouraging statements can help notoriety with feeling a more prominent identity worth and alleviation too. On the off chance that you notice your abettor is putting forth an fresh attempt on an extraordinary undertaking or on their appearance, you could offer a reassuring word or some recognition. They will presumably feel a lift in their soul and value you for taking note.

Offering your abettor an uplifting word can emphatically affect you, as well.

" Empowering explanations can be a doable framework for furthering correspondence, expressing appreciation, significant closeness, and multiple Congratulations Location certainty."

Ways of utilizing Inspiring proclamations

Be Legitimate

Independences who have encouraging statements as their affection words know each about bogus axioms, so be certain you're valid while drooling with your abettor . Be certain what you are talking about is coming from your heart.

You Look Perfect

As you both come of age, it can mean like no way ahead, indeed kinks and fresh pounds will generally proliferate as time passes. Search for the positive, and let it all out. Despite the fact that offering praise produces good sentiments, individualities constantly keep positive reflections down since they misestimate the huge worth they give their heirs.

On the off chance that you say," You look perfect!" you are really saying," I am still authentically drawn to you." As time passes, your mate will realize that you actually partake in their external as well as their inward nobility.

You are astonishing.

At the point when we decide to accompany notoriety for a really long time, formerly in a while we imagine that the other existent must supernaturally understand our study process. All effects considered, we could not hang out on the off chance that we did not consider the macrocosm of the other existent, correct? Now is the right time to express those considerations.

Tell your abettor ," you are astounding." What you're truly talking about is," you're a decent existent, and I love being with you."

Correspondence Them a Letter

Dispatch is an extraordinary system for conveying when you are in a rush, a commodity that stands out about getting an affection letter via the post office. Your abettor will be so astonished to get the letter from you. On the off chance that a letter appears to be overpowering, get them a fascinating card and compose an affable note outside.

Post a Note

Some of the time the stylish and most effective system for conveying the quantum you love your abettor is to use a sticky note and leave them a little communication about the quantum they mean to you. To get truly imaginative, you could post colorful notes looking like a heart or one further figure on the restroom reflection or the window of their vehicle.

Give Them a Holler

To insure you praise your uplifting statements to your abettor before others. Let them know what is right by you and what you truly appreciate. Try not to overstate it and cheapen your abettor , yet let others know how magnificent you suppose your abettor is will communicate their heart in similar innumerous ways. Therefore, do not be niggardly with the Commendation. This is an inconceivable system for filling your abettor 's affection tank.

Practice Encouraging statements all the time.

Anyhow, whether you aren't an encouraging statement individual, it's really smart to make uplifting statements an everyday propensity. While it presumably will not fluently fall into place, there are effects you can do to exercise offering uplifting statements all the time

Essay a pet name

Perhaps you can start every discussion with the pet name you have for your abettor . For example, you could say," Great morning, lovely" or" How are you, sweet pea?" These pet names might sound inelegant, yet for an encouraging individual, they can be exceptional.

Act naturally

Do whatever it takes not to come down on your tone or make statements that you do not feel. Simply allow yourself to be your real tone and offer what you value about your abettor .

Offer support

Uplifting statements do not simply need to be articulations of appreciation or praises — they can likewise zero in on words that amp your abettor . At the point when they express interest in a commodity or offer one of their objects with you, let them know that you have confidence in them and are backing them.

Heart-To-Heart

To build a more personal and commonly satisfying sincere relationship:

- Try to turn into a great heart-focused audience.

- Share appreciation and ardent appreciation.
- Little kindnesses procure huge profits.
- Keep your arrangements.
- Get a sense of ownership with your own fury.
- Praise your own and each other's triumphs.
- Fight the temptation to whine about your collaboration with your companions or family.

Create and keep up with strong and commonly settled upon standard procedures and rules.

1. Surrender individual space.

Assuming you have kids, particularly exceptionally small kids, you comprehend being willing to surrender individual space. At the point when they cry, you hold them. At the point when they're ravenous, you feed them. Thus it goes.

Presently clearly, we're not saying that at whatever point your accomplice makes a solicitation or interest, you promptly consent to fulfill it. We're discussing the mentality of eagerness to treat them with a similar nature of acknowledgment and cherishing as you would treat a baby or small kid.

At the point when they request something, truly consider what they are requesting as opposed to excusing it crazy since it doesn't match what you'd like at that time. What's more, since you're the two grown-ups and not parent and kid, at times such discussions are valuable open doors for figuring out how to utilize heart-focused tuning in (key number one) to arrange your disparities so they become commitments to your relationship as opposed to synergists of contentions.

Maybe this key has its most prominent handiness when every one of you might want to accomplish something else. Suppose you've chosen to head out to the films. Good gracious! You each need to see an alternate film. Expecting both of you are rehearsing the readiness to surrender individual space, you'll search for an inventive mutually beneficial arrangement.

You could settle on a third film you'd both like to see, or you could just have a pleasant supper out and skirt the film by and large. The key is adaptability... giving up when some piece of you (deciphering self image) might be ready and, as a matter of fact, situated to demand your direction of endeavoring to feel good or in charge.

How could you decide to do this? Since when you make imparting the wanting to your accomplice more significant than your own inclinations, you are putting aside installments in what we call your "Relationship Love Record."

This works with you both extending into a genuine sincere relationship whose money is cherishing, regarding, regarding, esteeming, euphoria and otherworldly important minutes.

2. Prize your accomplice.

A genuine relationship can be developed through working on valuing, which at its center includes you in moving into your heart and imparting to your accomplice your experience of their value. Entering the awareness of valuing not just moves you into your heart, it likewise opens the eyes of your heart! You'll see the internal excellence and completeness, or heavenliness, of your accomplice.

Furthermore, in that sacrosanct space, you'll likewise encounter your own. Unquestionably, this is one of the most immediate courses to imparting profoundly gorgeous minutes to your accomplice.

We should give it a shot. Go along with us briefly and shut your eyes... Center your mindfulness in your heart... bring your accomplice present there also... ponder the characteristics and approaches to being inside your accomplice that profoundly contact you.... most rouse you... What's present in your heart to impart to your accomplice?

3. Contact with adoration.

Heartily, liberally, energetically, pleasantly and sincerely share your adoration and friendship with your accomplice everyday. Actual touch is one of the manners in which you come into adoring reverberation with one another and orchestrate your energies.

No careless kiss on the cheek will at any point contact your own heart, not to mention your accomplice.

Clasping hands, putting your arm around your accomplice, rubbing their neck and shoulders, embracing, nestling, cuddling and delicate kisses give open doors to heart-to-heart and skin-to-skin association that add to a feeling of warmth, nurturance, prosperity and more profound encounters of shared closeness, cherishing and unity.

Contacting with adoration likewise helps keep the sentiment alive in your relationship. Open hearts are blissful hearts!

Chapter 5: Managing Conflict.

A contention in a relationship might be characterized as any sort of conflict, including a contention, or a continuous series of disagreements,for example, about how to burn through cash. Struggle can be very distressing, however it can likewise act to 'eliminate any confusion', surfacing issues that need discussion.Conflicts and conflicts might bring about us ending up being furious, and they may likewise emerge on the grounds that we have become irate about something different.

At work, we could attempt to control our outrage and try not to make statements we could lament. At home, tragically, we are substantially more liable to direct terrible sentiments toward others thus. There are likewise less inclined to be others around who can intercede, and conflicts subsequently rapidly raise in a way that probably won't occur at work.

This implies that contention in a relationship can quickly turn out to be exceptionally undesirable, and furthermore extremely private.

Five methodologies for overseeing struggle

1. **Contend or Battle,** the exemplary success/lose circumstance, where the strength and force of one individual wins the contention.
2. **Forswearing or Aversion,** where you imagine everything is good to go.
3. **Streamlining the Issue,** where you keep up with agreement on a superficial level, yet don't determine the contention.
4. **Split the difference or Discussion,** where both surrender something to make a center ground.
5. **Cooperation,** cooperating to make a common result.

These techniques are additionally pertinent to struggle in private and heartfelt connections.

Be that as it may, many individuals never get farther than forswearing, streamlining or battling. The issue with this, in any case, is that these are not long haul procedures to determine the issue. They are, best case scenario, hiding the faults, and this is unimaginable in a drawn out relationship (or rather, the relationship is probably not going to demonstrate long haul in the event that this is your picked approach).

The vitality in a relationship, hence, is to move past those three to think twice about, the best part is that joint effort.

In a split the difference, both of you quit any trace of something for a concurred mid-point arrangement

This is probably going to bring about an improved outcome than win/lose, yet it's not exactly a shared benefit. Since both of you have surrendered something, neither of you is probably going to be totally content with the result, which might prompt returning to the conversation again and again.

At the point when you team up, on the other hand, you cooperate to make a mutually beneficial arrangement, expanding on the contention.

It requires investment at the same time, seeing someone, merits the venture.

Moving towards joint effort

The unavoidable issue, obviously, is the way you can move towards cooperation, particularly in the event that you have previously settled an example of battling.

There are a couple of thoughts that will help:

1. Talk before you are irate and concur a methodology

Overseeing struggle requires a responsibility from both of you. Discuss how you might want to oversee conflicts, and furthermore concur that you will help each other to do that.

You might find it accommodating to discuss how you act when you are irate, and support each other to deal with that. For instance, on the off chance that one of you becomes furious rapidly, it could be useful for the other to propose holding on until some other time to talk.

2. Quit zeroing in on things that don't exactly make any difference

There is a maxim 'Don't perspire the little stuff'. It implies that you ought to zero in on what is important, and not stress over the things that truly don't make any difference so much.

Living with another person requires splitting the difference.

A decent spot to begin is with the 'little stuff': minor and oddball encroachments of your common 'rules'. These are much of the time not intentional, yet the aftereffect of your accomplice being drained, or absolutely getting diverted. It does not merit lashing out about these — until or except if they become standard, or a 'major thing' that truly irritates you.

Obviously assuming that they truly do become standard, or are truly aggravating you, it is worth focusing on them — yet pleasantly, not angrily

3. Try not to make individual assaults

At the point when you are irate, it is enticing to go after somebody such that you realize will hurt. Specifically, make an individual assault on their ethics, values or convictions.

Notwithstanding, staying away from this with your partner is significant.

Words said out of resentment might be difficult to neglect or excuse, whatever amount of you maintain that should do as such. All things considered, recall the 'rules of input' and spotlight on their way of behaving, and urgently, its impact on you.

4. Leave when you are furious

Start not talking about issues when you are furious. Offer something like:
"I can't talk currently, I'm simply excessively furious. Kindly we should discuss this some other time when I've quieted down."
Then leave, and go off somewhere to quiet down.

5. Try not to attempt to talk about troublesome things when you are drained or potentially eager

We are bound to be surly and troublesome when we are worn out or hungry. It is human instinct. Try not to have troublesome discussions at troublesome times. All things being equal, figure out an opportunity when you are both loose and agreeable, and the discussions are less inclined to grow into a contention. Certain individuals like to go out for a walk, and others carve out opportunities at home that are better: give things a shot and see what turns out best for you.

6. Continuously be ready to apologize

You might feel that you were justified. You might try and have been justified.

Being ready to apologize for the way that your accomplice feels, in any case, will go quite far towards guaranteeing that they believe they have been heard, and that you figure out their interests. This is particularly obvious if, in spite of your best expectations, you wound up yelling at one another.

Saying 'sorry' doesn't mean you need to acknowledge that you were off-base.

It implies saying that you are heartbroken that there was a conflict, and you are grieved that your accomplice is upset, and that you are focused on finding a way forward that works for you both.

7. Tune in and talk about

Be ready to pay attention to your accomplice. Try not to simply over and over make sense of your own perspective or you will wind up battling in the future. Building a split the difference or a cooperative arrangement requires genuine comprehension of what is essential to them, and why, and a conversation that imparts perspectives and insights usefully.

8. Try not to make suppositions

It is exceptionally simple to make presumptions about what your accomplice implied when they said x or y, or what is behind a specific piece of conduct.

Notwithstanding, attempt to oppose the enticement.

Rather than expecting, take a stab at asking them what they implied, or why they acted that way, or expressed out loud anything it was — and afterward truly stand by listening to what they say accordingly. This will assist you with seeing each other better.

Stay away from language that incites.

Correspondence doesn't generally come simple, whether it's with a better half or another person. In any case, it's critical to the general achievement and manageability of such organizations.

While certain individualities have no issue conducting their musts in an unmistakable and regardful manner, others might battle with respect to putting themselves out there and that can make keeping up with solid connections particularly testing.

There's a more critical regard to the colorful feathers of correspondence, how to deal with the manner in which you tune in and talk.

Advantages of Good Correspondence in a Relationship

Correspondence is the underpinning of any relationship," The degree to which each abettor is blessed at putting themselves out there, their conditions and their inclinations is the stylish sign of the good and satisfaction of the relationship"

As well as permitting you to communicate worries in a relationship, correspondence can help you resolve issues." Correspondence keeps couples in total agreement and feeling like they're dividing issues together as opposed to against each other," Successful correspondence also empowers cohorts to differ in useful, apprehensive ways.

Clear converse matters in any relationship. Many people could zero in erring on the nature of correspondence in close associations and have better norms of significant others than with family or companions, says Real, yet the significance of correspondence extends past that.

Certain capacities are important to keep up with open channels of correspondence that empower connections to flourish, whether with a significant other or another person.

" Each relationship requires correspondence — and the nature of that correspondence is an index of how satisfying the relationship is for the two individuals.

We as a whole need open correspondence in connections to connect holes despite a misconception, and to overcome our most worrisome difficulties." Open correspondence is the chine that holds up a relationship whether it's flourishing or under strain.

Great versus Unfortunate Correspondence in a Relationship

At its most essential, the discrepancy among great and unfortunate correspondence comes down to critical thinking and closeness. " Great correspondence explains issues and makes closeness between cohorts, while unfortunate correspondence strengthens issues and makes distance between cohorts".

As per every master, individualities display great correspondence when they:

- Focus and tune in while their abettor talks
- Pay attention to comprehend, as opposed to
- pay attention to answer authorize their abettor 's contemplations and sentiments(constantly by feting and rehashing back some of information changed)
- Seek explanation on some effects Comprehend, in any event, when their abettor has alternate points of view and suppositions
- Try not to speak loudly

In the interim, people with unfortunate correspondence propensities may:

- hamper

- Act in idle forceful ways

- Hold hard passions

- Pussyfoot around one another

- suspect or accept their abettor 's sentiments

- Hide issues down from plain view rather of work them out

- Contend further than formerly over a analogous subject

- Call their abettor names

- Convey intimidations

- Speak further loudly

The capacity to reliably conduct well seeing someone help with populating face difficulties and difficulties all the more gainfully, as indicated by Epstein." Sound correspondence helps couples-raise what's passing, remain cool-headed under pressure, use humor duly, apologize successfully and beget cohorts to feel appreciated and comprehended — in any event, during extremely distressing twinkles.

Feathers of Correspondence Styles

Scientists for the utmost part bunch correspondence into three classes tone- assured, frosty or forceful correspondence. Also, individualities use verbal correspondence to shoot dispatches to each other without words by any stretch of the imagination.

The following are four correspondence styles

1. Decisive Correspondence

This is the point at which you talk in an immediate way while conducting sympathy and a pining to suppose doubly about ways of addressing your musts, the specialists note." Decisive correspondence includes clear, befitting, regardful articulation," It comes from a position of simplicity about what an individual conditions.

2. Uninvolved Correspondence

Conveying latently implies you'll more frequently than not concede to others when now is the right time to go with a choice, says Real. Detached agents generally oblige others and stay down from inhibition." They're profoundly avoidant, will generally have an extremely lengthy circuit and are bound to leave a relationship rather than endorse their conditions inside the relationship".

3. Forceful correspondence

constantly includes going to clubs for your own freedoms at the adventure of maybe dismissing someone with different sentiments. An existent who resorts to this approach may presumably have a low capacity to bear close to home torture and will in general lash out further important of the time than others, says Real." At the point when they're heightened, they've a need to determine the contention right down, which as a rule brings about the circumstance raising since they are so over to speed in their own passions that they do not consider whether their abettor is professed or suitable to examine the issue," she says.

4. Verbal Correspondence

This kind of correspondence permits individualities to conduct data about their conditions, smarts, passions and points without exercising words. Verbal correspondence can be recovering and educational to couples when employed in non-latent forceful ways." Great verbal correspondence seems to be loosened up, reflecting non-verbal communication and eye to eye connection while talking," says Epstein. Still, it can take practice to get on specific prompts.

Tips On the stylish way to Work on Your Correspondence

The systems under can help you with figuring out how to all the more likely speak with your abettor .

Examine Your Correspondence Inclinations

Checking in with one another(beyond warmed twinkles) to probe requirements, musts and regions where you really want enhancement.

Questions like:

- How would you feel we conduct during disturbing twinkles?

- Do you feel appreciated and honored?

- While we are contending, what's it that you most anticipate from me?

- In the event that you could transfigure one thing about the manner in which I convey,
  What might it be?

- It seems like we get caught in teary patterns of crying at whatever point we contend.

- How would you suppose we each add to that uniqueness?

Plan a Common Relationship Meeting

You can utilize this assigned opportunity to rehearse great relational abilities while examining the week's difficulties and wins, supporting that discussions don't need to prompt struggle.

Chapter 6: Quality Time Together.

There is a distinction between getting to know each other and hanging out.

Essentially getting to know one another can be loaded up with things like working close to one another, finishing tasks simultaneously, perusing in a similar room as your accomplice is sitting in front of the television, and so forth.

Quality time is about carefully getting to know each other to show your appreciation and friendship for each other, and increasing association and closeness in your relationship. It implies not simply sitting in a similar room simultaneously, yet effectively deciding to set aside a few minutes for one another and for your relationship.

It is vital to make that qualification while taking a gander at the time enjoyed with your accomplice. When did you last get to know each other? Have you felt a separation from them, even while you're isolated with them? This could be on the grounds that the time you are spending together is programmed, or accidental. It isn't time saved explicitly to be with one another and center around your association.

So how might you invest significant quality energy?

The initial step: don't spend consistently together.

It sounds nonsensical, I know. In any case, despite the fact that we are social animals, enjoying the entire day with a similar individual (any individual) is an excess of time. You really want association and social cooperation, indeed, yet you additionally need space to depressurize, and to be without help from anyone else.

Furthermore, diminishing how much careless time spent together can assist with expanding the nature of the time you really do decide to spend together.

Clearly this is a lot harder in isolation. In the event that you live in a house with a yard you have more choices! However, in the event that you live in a loft or a little home it could appear to be difficult to figure out ways of spending opportunity separately.

Despite the fact that it's precarious, it's certainly feasible! Ways you can invest energy "separated" even around other people include:

- Take solo strolls. One accomplice can go for a stroll while the other stays at home, and afterward you can switch!
- Use earphones when in a similar room together. Make your very own headspace, in any event, while sharing actual space.
- Drape out in various regions of your home (regardless of whether they are still near one another). Perhaps one accomplice stays in the room while the other is in the parlor or the kitchen. Try not to go through your entire day in only one room, yet ensuring you have some alone time is critical!

The subsequent stage is: go with a reasonable settlement on when "quality together time" is.

It won't be the main time you spend together, so the two accomplices getting in total agreement about when the careful harmony ought to happen is vital to ensuring that time is quality time together.

Tell your accomplice you need to be deliberate about the time you're spending together. You can express something like: "I realize we go the entire day in a similar spot now at any rate, however I feel like it has caused us to neglect to focus on our association. Imagine a scenario in which we tried to have supper together, and center around being with each other during that feast, consistently."

You can pick quite a few activities together, yet discuss it ahead of time and settle on certain you're both understanding that this is the way you need to spend careful, deliberate time together.

How might you try and get to know each other?

Tragically, in isolation this is more enthusiastically than what we're utilized to. Typically if you had any desire to ensure you had quality time with your companion, you would most likely arrange a night out, or take off from the house! Presently, everything revolves around sorting out some way to separate between everyday space sharing, and quality time.

Fortunately, with quality time, what makes the biggest difference is the aim.

Most exercises can be "quality time" exercises assuming you do them carefully, and remain consistent with the goal that that time is for fellowship. These can include:

- Preparing a feast together. Arrange out a cookbook and go through it, and pick a recipe you are both amped up for. Regardless of whether one individual is a superior cook, take part in the entire cycle together. Remain present with one another.

- Peruse together. Not isolated books-pick something you both love (or something new!) and alternate perusing resoundingly to one another. Notice how you're feeling towards your accomplice, what the closeness feels like. At the point when you have a warm thought, express it without holding back rather than simply suspecting it!

- Sit together without screens. You don't have to design an "action" simply be together. Switch off your telephones, set aside your PCs, leave the television off. Sit together and talk.

- Take strolls together! At the point when you need to escape the house, walk connected at the hip with your accomplice around your area. Overlook the motivation to be on your telephone, and simply spend your walk zeroing in on your environmental elements and your accomplice.

- Play a game or do a riddle together. Find something imaginative or fun loving to do together!

Romance in sweet love

Being heartfelt is tied in with communicating adoration and devotion in a way that is purposeful, undeniable, and profoundly warm. It frequently includes sensational or enthusiastic motions, however more modest activities that demonstrate persevering through friendship can likewise be romantic.It by and large highlighted stories of knights, gallantry, and energy.

That is important for why sentiment today is frequently connected with over-the-top signals between darlings. "Being heartfelt includes making a feeling of enthusiasm, expectation, and energy inside a relationship,"

- Significant others needn't bother with being a particular character type; they can be loners, ambiverts, or outgoing people.
- A significant other, nonetheless, should be mindful, smart, willing, innovative, and kind of their accomplice's confidential and not-really secret longings."

Characteristics of a heartfelt individual:

1.Affectionate

Most importantly, a heartfelt individual is ready to routinely show the amount they love and revere the object of their friendship. They could consistently offer little shows of friendship, whether that is through demonstrations of service,words of assertion, or other sweet motions.

Whether you bring your accomplice an adoration-filled mug of espresso every morning, foam each other's backs in the shower, or appreciate clasping hands as you walk, genuine sentiment is tied in with showing your adoration for one another in predictable, significant ways. "Steady shows of significant consideration (whether it's kissing, little symbolic gifts, contact, or saying romantic things') 'can keep a heartfelt state of mind alive consistently."

2.Thoughtful

The most heartfelt of accomplices are the people who are aware of their life partner's requirements and wants in enthusiastic, smart ways. "The main propensity shift to make if attempting to turn out to be more heartfelt is mindfulness. Assuming you have checked out what your accomplice needs and needs, you can make unconstrained shocks and long haul heartfelt examples that will forever excite your accomplice."

3.Dedicated

Critically, a heartfelt individual doesn't simply offer a lot of gifts and romantic things with no genuine importance behind them. An enormous piece of what makes a person or thing heartfelt is the possibility that the adoration and enthusiasm they offer is steadfast and persevering, and it's extraordinarily proposed to a particular individual. That is which isolates a heartfelt individual from a tease: the force, life span, and particularity of their sentiments.

That is the reason the most heartfelt discourses or love letters model, are frequently profoundly customized: "For a long-term love, you need to discuss recollections, beating obstructions together, what made you become hopelessly enamored at first, why you actually love them today, and what you find from here on out,"

4.A inclination for enormous motions

The first idea of sentiment came from accounts of the gallant deeds of knights able to set out their lives for affection. In current times, sensational motions are as yet connected with sentiment: making a trip significant distances to shock the individual you love, proposing before a major horde of individuals, or even just discussing your future together right off the bat in a relationship.

5.Sentimental

Heartfelt individuals could likewise explicitly depict their affection for somebody in profoundly nostalgic, grandiose, or amazing terms, for example, portraying their darlings as "perfect partners," discussing how destiny united them, or pronouncing that their adoration will last them to the grave and then some. They might tend to glorify their accomplice or their relationship too, which may not precisely be a solid inclination, regardless of its sentimentalism.

6 .Present

On the other hand, not every person will think about clearing signals and beyond ludicrous announcements of affection to be heartfelt. Once in a while being a heartfelt individual is just about being profoundly present, warm, and loving with your accomplice in the everyday minutes.

" Huge gifts and pivotal excursions are reaching, champion twinkles in a relationship,"

7.Consistent

Being a heartfelt individual method establishing a vibe of warm love and enthusiasm all year, not simply on extraordinary events like Valentine's Day or somebody's birthday, Masculine brings up.

"A certified better half tends to 'date' [their] enormous other all through the relationship as opposed to committing genuine energy to two or three brand name dates every month or year,"

ways of being heartfelt.

Work on having more slow, more genuinely associated sex.

- Plan a heartfelt escape with your accomplice through and through, so they don't need to ponder any of the arranging subtleties.

- Continuously kiss your accomplice great morning, great evening, hi, and farewell.

- Come up from behind your accomplice while they're following through with something and fold your arms over them.

- Hold your accomplice's hand, or put your arm around them openly.

- Watch heartfelt films together, and afterward begin acquiring the best lines into how you converse with your accomplice.

- Watch heartfelt motion pictures together, and afterward begin getting the best lines into how you converse with your accomplice.

- While they're conversing with you, truly tune in — set aside any tech, visually connect, and completely take part in the discussion.

- Kiss your accomplice in puts other than on the lips: Attempt their brow, back of the hand, or shoulder.

- Get innovative with how you express your affection: Use allegories, reference past recollections, and go past "I love you."

Chapter 7: Allow Your Partner to Influence You.

Inviting your accomplice's feedback and sentiments — tolerating impact — is a strong methodology for creating further association, regard, and confidence in your relationship. Figuring out how to acknowledge impact is tied in with tracking down ways of saying "OK" to each other, which I love.

As you embrace a more delicate, humble position, it leaves space for interest — and, surprisingly, amazing results that you may in all likelihood never have anticipated from your relationship with your accomplice.

Be that as it may, figuring out how to acknowledge impact doesn't simply occur. It requires turning towards your accomplice and freeing yourself dependent upon them with a goal. What's more, now and again, while you're beginning,

it could require a couple of standard procedures.

Perhaps this seems to be thinking of a signal:a safe-expression of sorts that permits your accomplice to convey how they don't feel they're being heard or regarded.

"In light of everything, I have zero faith in most men — or people in general — to be antagonistic or mean or discourteous".

However, correspondence breakdowns happen constantly — not a solitary one of us is resistant to this. Assuming you feel that your accomplice is being those things, concur with each other on a sign.

Several have an expression or flag they can use to assist each other better with tolerating influence: But what works for one couple may not work for another.
Perhaps it's a break signal, one that says,
"Hang on. I don't feel like you're available to tolerate my impact at the present time. I believe you should pause and hear me."

Or on the other hand maybe your sign seems to be a delicate word: like,
"Umm… You're doing that thing you do" or,
"Could we at any point make a stride back so we can both have input?"
Involving a word or an expression in this manner can prompt an opening, an alternate result.

Driving with weakness can function admirably, too: Phrases such as, "I don't feel like I'm being heard at the present time" or, "I really want you to tune in" assist us with communicating the requirement for sympathy, delicacy, and adoring empathy.

Finding what will work in your relationship is really significant: In the event that you can do that, you'll be well headed to sharing impact and tolerating impact — to the extraordinary advantage of your relationship.

When you comprehend the worth and effect of tolerating impact in your relationship, we're certain you'll need to deal with making it a piece of your coexistence immediately. In any case, similar to anything, figuring out how to do that requires some investment.

Appreciation and gratitude.

We have a ton of affection in our souls for the notable individuals in our lives. We favor them as we see them giggle, and trust that the best things become a piece of their excursion.

It's all superb, yet the majority of it is inside us. How frequently do we effectively offer thanks to individuals nearest to us for every one of the manners in which they make our life lovely?

At the point when somebody is unfamiliar to us, an accomplice, companion, or relative, being amped up for every one of the beneficial things about them is simple. We look for the exceptional pieces of their character and are quick to know them more.

Be that as it may, over the long haul, and they become a customary piece of our lives, we begin to loosen, decreasing the work, care, and consideration we used to give them.

To have delightful, satisfying, major areas of strength for and, we should do the best for our friends and family, and what is preferred far over applying the infinitesimal thankful course of appreciation?

These are ways Of utilizing Appreciation and Appreciation to Develop Further Connections

1. Offer gratitude for doing what they "ought to do"
2. Esteem their dreams and characteristics
3. Regard their time
4. Be appreciative for their presence
5. Be predictable

1. Offer thanks for doing what they "should do"

Your accomplice, your parents, or your companion, should treat you well, support you, and be adoring towards you, yet that doesn't reduce the significance of what they do.

At the point when your cherished one gets you water, helps you out with a task, pays attention to your viewpoints, or strolls to the supermarket with you, it is fundamental to feel thankful for their presence and exertion.

In every last manner that they make your life simpler and better, there should be appreciation, and one that is valid. Saying an aloof "much appreciated" won't bring the train back home.

Pause for a minute to genuinely see the value in every one of the parts where they are available in your life and cause them to feel unique for ordinary things.

2. Value their fantasies and characteristics

We as a whole have our unusual characteristics, the things that recognize us and give a remarkable flavor to our character.

Furthermore, we as a whole have dreams that we believe that others should put stock in. What are the weird methods of your loved ones? What are their fantasies? Intentionally value what makes them remarkable and invigorated.

Is it the manner in which they sniffle? Or on the other hand the manner in which they recount stories? Might it be said that they are fixated on vehicles? Do they fantasize about opening up a library or taking on 100 canines?

We should earnestly praise the astonishing things about them and let them in on how great they are.

3. Esteem their time

A significant number of our friends and family invest a great deal of energy with us. We miss the ones that don't, however , don't see the value in the ones that do. On second thought, it's a seriously extraordinary gift.

We should accept this second to see the value in how valuable the endowment of their time is. Their accessibility to us is an honor and we should treat it that way.

In the event that they have decided to be with us for the greater part of their days, it's an extremely valuable present. How about we appreciate the time that our nearby ones eagerly share with us.

4. Be thankful for their presence

This is a speedy update that life is unusual. We should be careful to not underestimate our friends and family and be perpetually accessible. There is no conviction that what we have now will be with us in the entire days to come.

Quite a few variables can become an integral factor and change what is happening. Consistently, we should continue to offer genuine thanks for individuals present in our lives and recognize that it wouldn't be entirely ideal without them.

5. Be reliable

Now that we've drilled down four fundamental ways of involving appreciation for building more grounded connections, we should rehearse this well. Consistency is critical assuming we wish to get results.

As appreciation journaling ought to be done day to day to notice its best effects, offering thanks to our friends and family ought to likewise be rehearsed determinedly. How about we be committed to our connections and give our heart to building them as unequivocally as could be expected.

Along these lines, you are right there. These are a few different ways that appreciation can be utilized to develop further connections. At the point when we're not careful, we take the main ever-present pieces of our lives for granted. We should improve and rehearse appreciation for the easily overlooked details and dear individuals to carry on with a genuinely supernatural life!

Chapter 8: Continuous Growth.

Trust your accomplice by confiding in yourself first. Be transparent with your accomplice by being transparent with yourself first. Developing a solid relationship is a continuous experience -- requiring fun loving nature, inventiveness, and responsibility.

Numerous connections and relationships frequently come up short on account of how two individuals become together. The relationship either develops into adoration and congruity - or it develops into doubt, question, disdain - in the end prompting a separation or separation.

Further developing our relationship is a continuous experience, in light of the fact that a hot, energizing relationship takes fun loving nature, imagination, responsibility and an open heart.

As a shrewd man once said, you won't ever arrive at your maximum capacity in the event that you don't open your heart.

keep your relationship developing by:

1) Trust

Nothing damages and breaks a relationship as fast as untrustworthiness. At the point when trust is lost it propels ways of behaving like analysis, dismissal, and desirously.

Genuineness and trust are the most noteworthy types of closeness. In the event that you lie once, every one of your bits of insight can become problematic. At the point when you tell the truth, you produce legit activities and responses.

2) Want

Want fills in as the association among adoration and sex.

The craving we feel for the other individual means that the exuberance and immediacy in our lives and in our relationship.

Want is to cherish what wood is for fire. Want without affection can bring about a condition of yearning and destitution.

3) Love

A piece of human love is puzzling, mysterious, free streaming, and once in a while outside of our reach.

Love is a word that covers different sentiments. Love is an inclination. On one hand it tends to be an outright pleasure, while then again it very well may be unadulterated graciousness.

Love uncovers our capability to see, feel, contact, and smell, what we've won't ever dream of.

How we experience love is a decision. It can appear suddenly and feel like that individual was made explicitly for us.

Cherishing each other means tolerating each other precisely as they are. You have a deep understanding of the individual and welcome everything. You have seen every one of their qualities regardless need to be a piece of their life.

Mature love is something other than a warm inclination; it's a lifestyle - like making an inestimable show-stopper. It requires acknowledgment, persistence, or more all, everyday practice.

4) Closeness

One of the main opinions of human love is closeness, since quite possibly the most significant articulation signifies, "in-to-me-see."

Closeness is being tolerating and being defenseless. Closeness doesn't mean experiencing passionate feelings in the regular feeling of heartfelt fascination, yet arising in adoration by understanding what compels you and your accomplice to extend and become together.

5) Correspondence

Open, legit correspondence ought to be essential for each sound relationship.

Significant discussions ought not be put off, yet neither would it be advisable for them they be started during abnormal or unseemly times. Raising room issues during a vacation party isn't the most ideal spot to have such a conversation.

Profound discussions require profound tuning in. Being straightforward when you feel irate is difficult, however on the off chance that what you're talking about isn't correct, then, at that point, nothing genuine is being shared.

Going into a discussion with a plan might prompt botched open doors for association, more profound comprehension of your accomplice, and their explanations behind how they approach specific circumstances.

The more appended you are to the result the more frustrated you'll be.

6) Mindfulness

The manner in which you view your assets, suppositions, feelings, and appearance is your single most significant perspective on the real world. Try not to leave yourself.

Get a sense of ownership with your activities and development by giving first concern to the physical, close to home, mental, and profound parts of your life.

The manner in which we characterize ourselves is a decision. Our decision each second.

At the point when you know what your identity is, you don't permit others to characterize you.

At the point when you disregard to take adoring consideration of yourself - - (by overlooking your own sentiments, and making a decision about yourself) you wind up feeling penniless and unreliable.

This feeds the anxiety toward losing your accomplice or losing yourself.
Dread shuts the heart. Love opens it. Sound self esteem begins by figuring out how to be available and aware of your sentiments - - instead of proceeding to keep away from them.

7) Opportunity

Being seeing someone connectedness and aloneness. It's an incredible inclination when you can keep up with your opportunity and freedom while likewise remaining profoundly associated with your accomplice.

A relationship established in dread based feelings, for example, desire, outrage, uncertainty, tension and possession can raise question, doubt, and poverty.

Trust your accomplice by confiding in yourself first. Be transparent with your accomplice by being transparent with yourself first.

Developing a sound relationship is a continuous experience - - requiring fun loving nature, inventiveness, and responsibility.

Cherishing life and death.

Cherishing. The word indeed has the sound of delicacy, of holding dear, of warmth toward one further coming from the spirit.

Valuing is over all additional love, still one can adore without esteeming. Valuing is a lifted up type of adoration, the most noteworthy, noblest, deepest inclination one existent can have for another. Esteeming is an adoration for the other that has come to development, to completion. It's a holding of the physical, yet of unearthly, profound and scholarly aspects partook just the same as the other.Cherishing requires the sharing of reality together, and a seasoning of the relationship as it's developed, restored and celebrated day to day.

One who loves sees another not as an expansion of tone but rather as an extraordinary, constantly getting, pleasurable existence.

The existent who loves encompasses one further with a cloak of poise and regard, ending from judgment and redundancy.That individual establishes a climate so defended the other can partake their deepest sentiments, dreams, bummers or palms unafraid of imputation.
There's space for botches without discipline, indeed huge bones, for botches are viewed as pivotal for the most common way of getting. What is further, there's constant forgiveness.

The existent who values likewise finds in the other his veritably own print humanness and the phenomenon of life. He treats the other with an analogous delicacy, fidelity and awe as he'd a child sprat. His adoration is not requesting, nor does it calculate upon legality or value. Neither does it keep track of who is winning.

The person who appreciates really wants to associate with the other, to encounter that existent's most profound internal identity and to partake, accordingly, his own. He encounters explosions of affection coming from the tone nearly outside. He communicates that affection through demonstrations of delicacy, appreciation and commitment, and he at any point confirms the other's presence and worth. His steady fellowship and evidence makes the valued one feel a tranquility, a satisfaction, that comes from constantly being unobtrusively guaranteed of the other's affection.

One lady portrays her hassles in treasuring and being loved in her marriage. Agitating her significant other, she says" I truly like him a ton. He is great each round. He wears his sentiments on his sleeves and he cries before me.

" He is intriguing. He has giggly effects that make me chuckle. I feel more when he connects with me and when I put my head on his shoulder.

" He is an old chum. He understands me better than anybody. What is further, I can perceive he prefers me. In some cases it's in the manner in which he discusses me when I am not there. He tells me constantly that he values me for what I have done and that he adores me. He is likewise legal with me. I can trust him.

" At times he has a particular total search in his eyes that supports me inside-it finishes me off. " He is a little fat and he is rehearsing extremes at the present time. There are exacerbating effects about the two of us, still we have figured out how to neglect them.

" He means quite a bit to me. I really want him. There is nothing on earth I wouldn't do for him. He is indelible to my heart. At the point when he is missing, I miss his presence. It resembles a major void when he is not with me. I do not believe that he should vanish. It cheers me up to have him around.

" Says someone differently regarding couples and loving." You can tell, in any event, when you do not realize others well, whether they esteem one another."

For most outrageous couples, treasuring is a charge-a condition unattained still quite close. To foster one's capability to value, an existent should arrive at the outside to see the weak tone and to communicate that tone in delicate, sustaining and engaging ways.

Valuing requires surrendering the strength, brutality and anxiety that constantly come from fasting on all that over individualities in one's day to day actuality. What is further, it requires clearing close to home space inside oneself, to consider and to see the value in the precious and necessary worth of a friend or family member.

To appreciate, one must likewise arrive at beyond tone to avow through demonstrations of affection the worth of the other. Treasuring requires turning out to be all the more profoundly involved, more helpless, more responsive, seriously participating and further cozy.

Couples who love, obviously, comprehend that perfectly.

What Not to Do.

Self-fault or retribution

Quit Rebuffing YOUR Abettor Everybody has encountered results in their lives- breaks as a sprat, being disregarded working, advanced insurance payments after an bus collision.

Be that as it may, there's one spot discipline will not ever have a place in your relationship. Feting rebuffing conduct in a relationship is an advanced precedent than any time in recent memory in our separated and socially confined world.

We're investing decreasingly more energy at home with our cohorts, and it's normal for this to prompt a lot of dissatisfaction and indeed correspondence issues as we explore this new geography. Being rebuffed seeing someone not the same as the commonplace contentions or clashes two or three appearances. It's a significant relationship issue and should be tended to right down.

DIscipline in connections

Discipline in connections is the point at which one abettor designedly attempts to beget the other to really lament an exertion or conduct that they expostulate to. While you are rebuffing your abettor , you need to show them a" illustration" about a commodity they did with the thing that they won't repeat the experience from then on out.

There are numerous feathers of rebuffing conduct in a relationship. Obviously, factual maltreatment should Norway be endured. In any case, discipline constantly comes in fresh unpretentious structures.

The vast maturity perceives the quiet treatment- yet it's really a type of discipline. Rejecting fondness or closeness can be employed as discipline. Resting on the chesterfield president or staying down from your abettor is clearly a rebuffing conduct, as is designedly dismembering your abettor - for case, by making them late or" neglecting" to negotiate commodity they inquired.

At the point when we blow up seeing someone, truly comes from a position of dread- dread that a person or thing is not working out as anticipated. Our abecedarian mortal demand for conviction is not being satisfied, so we respond by demanding to recover control of the circumstance. What is further, one of the most extensively honored- and likewise generally harming- ways that we do that's by rebuffing notoriety in a relationship.

What happens when there's rebuffing conduct in a relationship?

Discipline is a commodity contrary to correspondence, which is the reason it's so harmful to connections. As opposed to getting to the core of the issue and managing it, the absence of correspondence energies detachment and pushes you vastly further separated. Therefore, this causes you to feel indeed less in charge.

At the point when you begin to brush-off your abettor , you risk making a profound degree of injury. There's no adoration in discipline- just hurt, agony and casualness that prompts

- **Hopelessness**

Being rebuffed seeing someone the two cohorts- including the one doing the rebuffing- sense significantly more alone and more misgauge .

- ### **Difference**

Rebuffing conduct in a relationship constantly shows an irregularity as one abettor holds control over the other. You can not authentically fill in as a group when there's a power irregularity along these lines.

- ### **Absence of trust**

When discipline in connections is employed again and again, there can be a serious break in trust, so that whether or not both of you stay in the relationship, there will be a gigantic close to home, internal and, unexpectedly, profound gap.

- ### **Counter**

Connections that application discipline as a device can stall out in a pattern of reprisal- one abettor feels they were rebuffed unjustifiably and subsequently rebuffs their abettor accordingly. Try not to stall out in this retaliatory illustration.

The abettor being rebuffed seeing someone set up a wall to shield themselves from persisting through further agony. In any case, what's the other option? How would you communicate your failure and guarantee that your abettor earnings from the experience? It boils down to one crucial fixing- joy.

Why does betrayal hurt so profoundly?

Treacheries can genuinely affect an individual. They take many structures and occur for different reasons, however they share a central trait - they can pass on serious close to home scars and injury to the people who have been deceived.

The underlying response to treachery differs. A few people will, from the start, feel shocked and confused, while others will experience quick rage or trouble. We all are unique, and we respond to terrible and harmful circumstances in our own specific manners.

Notwithstanding, the vast majority will, sooner or later, experience an absence of trust toward the individual who deceived them. While this is an issue that can be survived, it can really harm a relationship on the off chance that accomplices don't figure out how to determine this issue.

That is quite possibly the main motivation why disloyalty is so hard to survive. Introductory close to home responses die down, while an absence of trust waits. Also, trust can be incredibly hard to modify.

Side effects Of Treachery

It can fluctuate for everybody, influencing both physical and psychological wellness because of a critical selling out, especially by somebody they trusted or relied on.

1. **Profound trouble:** Serious feelings like shock, outrage, misery, hurt, and disarray are normal following a treachery. These feelings can be overpowering and hard to make due, prompting inner strife and insecurity.

2. **Nervousness and dread:** The sold out individual might encounter tension, dread, or even frenzy because of the double-crossing. This can appear as a consistent condition of stress, hypervigilance, or a staggering feeling of dread toward additional treachery.

3. **Misery:** Delayed sensations of sadness and gloom can be indications of wretchedness following double-crossing injury. This might bring about a deficiency of interest in exercises once delighted in, changes in hunger or rest examples, and trouble focusing or deciding, causing a change in your emotional wellness.

4. **Meddling contemplations and rumination:** Treachery injury can prompt consistent considerations about the double-crossing, frequently joined by a powerful urge to comprehend the reason why it worked out. This can bring about rumination, where the individual becomes distracted with the selling out and experiences issues zeroing in on different parts of their life.

5. **Relationship issues:** Trust is in many cases broken following a disloyalty, which can prompt troubles in framing new connections or keeping up with existing ones. The sold out accomplice might be more watched, less open, or excessively dubious of others' aims.

6. **Confidence and self-esteem:** Disloyalty injury can leave the singular scrutinizing their own value and worth. They might encounter deep-seated insecurities,

self-fault, or self-question, which can additionally add to their profound misery.

7. **Rest aggravations:** Rest issues like sleep deprivation, bad dreams, or fretful rest can be side effects of treachery injury. The profound and mental pressure can make it challenging to unwind and nod off or prompt bad dreams connected with the treachery.

8. **Actual side effects**: The pressure of treachery injury can influence actual wellbeing by appearing as actual side effects, including migraines, stomach related issues, muscle strain, or a general sensation of being unwell.

9. **Separation and withdrawal:** Trying to shield themselves from additional hurt, the double-crossed may pull out from social communications, stay away from circumstances that help them to remember

the disloyalty, or seclude themselves from companions

Why Selling Out So Agonizing?

Selling out in a heartfelt connection can make you overthink your whole relationship. It can permit weakness to crawl into your relationship with your accomplice, which is an individual bond remembered to be sufficiently able to endure any test.

Unreliable Connection

Drawing on the connection hypothesis, we can more readily comprehend the aggravation of selling out injury and how our connection styles impact our profound reactions and survival methods. On the off chance that either accomplice has encountered selling out or broken trust before throughout everyday life, this recurrent treachery can have significant impacts mentally.

The first injury was horrendous and can appear in a wide range of ways.

For example, an individual who experienced actual maltreatment by somebody during youth might have fostered a restless connection style bringing about huge trust issues in connections.

The tensely joined accomplice fears dismissal and deserting and has been known to likewise expect double-crossing.

Suppose that this specific individual has not recently participated in treatment or self-awareness work. So presently, they've been double-crossed by their accomplice for someone else.

The particular trust issues established in their young life reemerge, and their profound response is to sit down in the fetal situation in bed throughout the following few days, frozen.

This experience of rehash treachery injury can be both pulverizing and excruciating.

Rehashed examples of double-crossing can compound existing close to home injuries and bring up a pattern of self-issue and weakness, making intricacies in heartfelt connections and then some.

This can make it progressively provoking for people to break liberated from the examples of doubt and dread that have been imbued in their mind.

Trust Is Broken

Contingent upon the individual, disloyalties are difficult for different reasons. Notwithstanding, double-crossing in connections normally harms us since we frequently feel that our accomplice, who should be nearest to us, acted against us and presented us to torment through their activities.

Also, for that reason double-crossing harms to such an extent. Where there was conviction, there is currently vulnerability. Where there was understanding, there is currently misconstruing. Also, where there was conviction, there is currently a question. Also, that damages. As trust disintegrates, people might end up addressing their accomplice's genuineness as well as their own value and capacity to keep up with sound connections. This can prompt sensations of disconnection, despair, and being caught in a pattern of selling out and torment.

Regardless of the infringement of trust you or your accomplice have encountered, it tends to be extremely challenging to determine and survive. Double-crossing injury can be genuinely depleting and destroying.

Be that as it may, everybody has their faults. Committing errors doesn't mean we don't cherish our accomplices, we don't see the value in them, or we would rather not accompany them.

At Turn, we view adoration as an action word. Is it true that you are being adored toward your accomplice? Occasionally for individual reasons, we may not feel fit for giving and getting love. Life challenges emerge and can here and there bring a gigantic measure of dread, restless sentiments, and discouragement. Not feeling cherished doesn't pardon deceiving our accomplices. Openness is of the utmost importance. It is your obligation to share how you feel with one another so assumptions are sensible.

Botches occur. How we manage those errors is what we can use to show our accomplices exactly the amount we care about them. So indeed, you can adore your accomplice and double-cross them. Or then again be adored and feel deceived. On the off chance that it works out, it's essential to show them the amount you give it a second thought and assume liability. Do what's an option for you to make things right.

Disloyalty is a complicated and excruciating experience that can lastingly affect people and connections. However there is certainly not a generally acknowledged model for the phases of disloyalty in private connections, numerous clinicians and relationship specialists propose different structures to assist with grasping the cycle. Here is one such structure that separates treachery into stages:

5 Phases Of Selling out

- **Revelation:** This is the underlying stage when the double-crossed individual becomes mindful. It is frequently portrayed by shock, mistrust, and disarray as the singular attempts to deal with the data and get a handle on what has occurred.

- **Personal commotion:** In this stage, the deceived individual encounters an out of control thrill ride of feelings, including outrage, hurt, and gloom. It's normal for people to feel genuinely wrecked and to sway between various feelings as they endeavor to adapt to the disloyalty. During this stage, in the event that the double-crossed individual had a comparable past injury, the feelings, and their precariousness are enhanced.

- **Importance making:** During this stage, the deceived individual begins to dissect the selling out trying to comprehend the reason why it worked out. They might scrutinize their own decisions, the activities of the traitor, and the conditions encompassing the disloyalty. This stage can include a lot of contemplation and self-reflection.

- **Reconstructing:** In this stage, the double-crossed accomplice concludes whether they need to fix the relationship or continue on. Assuming they decide to chip away at the relationship, they will probably lay out new limits, participate in open correspondence with the double-crosser, and look for proficient assistance in the event that they haven't as of now. In the event that they choose to continue on, they might begin to make another existence without the double-crosser, zeroing in on their own mending cycle and self-improvement.

- **Acknowledgment and mending:** This last stage includes grappling with the treachery and discovering a feeling of conclusion. The deceived individual figures out how to pardon, either to reestablish the relationship or to give up and push ahead. This stage is set apart by revamping trust, self-awareness and a recently discovered association with self and others.

It's critical to take note that these stages are not direct, and people might move to and fro between them as they process the demonstration of disloyalty. Moreover, the span and force of each stage can change contingent upon the idea of the demonstration of treachery and the singular's strategies for dealing with hardship or stress.

How Would You Manage Treachery In A Relationship?

Being sold out is sufficiently hard, however managing and defeating relationship treachery can be much more challenging to do.

There is no set rundown of decides that will assist you with beating disloyalty in your relationship quicker or better, yet here are a few hints that could be useful to you have sound connections and manage treachery somewhat more without any problem:

- Name and embrace the feelings you're feeling, as recognizing how you feel is the most vital move toward recuperation.

- Try not to want to clear up your affections for anybody or to justify them.
- Oppose from the possible longing to fight back to treachery.
- Take as the need might arise to find some peace with your relationship disloyalty.
- Evaluate the disloyalty and endeavor to reveal the potential explanations for it.
- Attempt to tranquilly examine the selling out with your accomplice and pay attention to their side.
- Take your contemplations and sentiments to a held proficient person to help you.
- Realize that you don't need to remain. Assuming that the selling out is excessively harmful to you, you can pursue handling what to do, and if the choice to leave is where you end up, that is a legitimate choice. Frequently when kids, cash, and different variables are involved, it is vital to give yourself an opportunity to comprehend what occurred and why it worked out so you can continue on without conveying extra stuff.

Jealousy

Desire can be a strong and difficult inclination, and this pessimistic inclination can cut off practically any friendship. Whenever left untreated, envy can make an extremely durable wedge among you and your accomplice, while adversely influencing future connections.

Where Does Desire Come From?

Desire essentially emerges from instability inside oneself and not confiding in your accomplice.

Jealousy and envy are comparative, as a matter of fact. Be that as it may, envy includes a feeling of possessiveness and qualification while a jealous individual wants what someone else has for their assets, positions, honors or their identity personally (their looks).

An envious individual hangs on firmly to what they as of now have-as a rule their better half to fend others from taking this individual off.

At the point when jealousy and desire gain out of influence, it very well may be exceptionally damaging.

How To Move Past Desire?

Desire in a relationship can be recuperated. Two or three arrangements with envy and different contentions is crucial to their prosperity.
Transparently discussing your thoughts about being shaky or dubious in your relationship starts the discussion.

Recollect

- Talk from your heart
- Try not to legitimize your activities,
- Try not to make allegations
- Try not to be fierce

Discussing your interests, your questions and your desires is alright. View this season of pressure as a chance for open correspondence and extension of understanding for the two accomplices.

Tame Your Creative mind

It is astonishing that something that gets going in our creative mind can before long start wild and cause such annihilating harm. Creative mind develops envy like seeds, compost, sun and water develop your nursery.

Perceive the negative stories and steady self-talk. Try not to make a huge deal about things by going over them consistently to you. Simply envision all things being equal, having the option to do everything that fulfills you as opposed to having that large number of pessimistic considerations and feelings going around inside your head.

Envision not fixating and stress over each seemingly insignificant detail.
You ought to likewise take the best of luck at those things that trigger your envy. Cautiously

consider the bazaar-like circumstances you have envisioned about your accomplice and what genuine proof you need to approve them.

Desire knows no judicious reasoning and it has not a great explanation. Do a rude awakening by surveying your fanatical contemplations with what you really know or have seen. Drop considerations of intrigue and supplant them with genuine realities.

Besides, even a little conflict can ignite a monstrous battle due to desire. Assuming your own uncertainty or low mental self portrait makes you think gravely about yourself, you frequently start to consider what your better half finds in you.

It is basic to deal with working on yourself as a person to be an entire and equivalent accomplice in your relationship.
Rather than getting enveloped with circumstances in which you have no control over, attempt a pressure diminishing way of life.

Engage in gatherings and exercises that help you have a positive outlook on yourself. Center around your assets. Furthermore, definitely, have more than one companion.

How To Relinquish The Past?

Continually going over adverse occasions of the past denies you of the present and causes you to feel terrible. It is vital to trust and have total confidence in your accomplice to forestall envious inclinations toward them.

Consider your accomplice and every day to be a new beginning and chance to become together, instead of reiterating and remembering your previous encounters of uncertainty and depression.

It's essential to comprehend that envy is a feeling that can torture the one you care generally about. Envy might in fact turn out to be all things considered a fixation, as a matter of fact. The negligence that you put on that individual through your envious uncertainties is as genuine to them as your sensations of being caught in your own jail of uncertainty.

Recognize that what you most apprehension - your accomplice leaving you - is precisely the exact thing you are sustaining with your damaging and possessive examples.

Think about the results of your puncturing uncertainties. Acknowledge desire isn't just disastrous yet a forlorn spot to be.

How Would I Deal with A Desirous Accomplice?

Having an envious accomplice can debilitate. There is just such a lot of possessiveness, control and addressing you can take. There are things you can do to energize a better relationship. The following are a couple of tips:

- Pay attention to your cooperate with new ears to hear their interests in general

- Assuming you realize specific ways of behaving trigger your accomplice's desire, change them if possible

- Bring up what you most value about the person in question, and deal consolation that you are focused on the relationship

- Let your accomplice know what you most need in your relationship. Try not to simply say, "I believe that you should quit being envious!"

Remember it takes the two individuals to make an incredible relationship. Notwithstanding, in the event that your accomplice isn't willing to change or find support, you can make changes in yourself that will enormously affect your life to improve things.

CONCLUSION

In conclusion"Fundamental Assumption for Strong Relationship," it's obvious that the profoundly imbued suspicions and convictions we hold structure the bedrock whereupon our associations flourish or waver. Through nuanced investigations and functional techniques, this story enlightens the basic underpinnings that shape persevering, flourishing connections.

Each page of this book reverberates as a song of praise, calling people to intentionally develop a system of trust, compassion, and immovable responsibility. It's a convincing update that suppositions are not simple quiet convictions but rather strong, dynamic specialists that reinvigorate each collaboration and choice inside a relationship.

The account urges perusers to reconsider these suppositions, motivating them to embrace an ethos of figuring out, regard, and commonality as they navigate the delightful, unpredictable landscape of organization. It allures them to cultivate a climate where love, compassion, and getting through association are establishments as opposed to an idea in retrospect.

As perusers close the last section, they are called to set out on a groundbreaking excursion, committed to developing presumptions that honor and treasure the pith of their accomplices and the sacredness of their connections. It's a mixing call to write a story of significant love, versatility, and faithful help — a future portrayed by cognizant, significant suspicions that reinvigorate their common process.

On the whole, "Fundamental Assumption for Strong Relationship" arises as an aide as well as an enthusiastic buddy, rousing people to challenge, stir, and eventually shape a future grounded in the faithful strength of conscious, engaging suspicions — a future secured in the wonderful ethos of persevering, flourishing adoration.

Embrace the groundbreaking force of suspicions. Decorate your relationship with an ethos of trust and significant association.

Set out to record your noteworthy story established in the ethos of steady, cognizant, and significant suspicions.